IMOGENE KING

A Conceptual Framework for Nursing

Christina L. Sieloff Evans

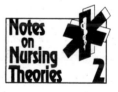

Notes on Nursing Theories 2

SAGE PUBLICATIONS
The International Professional Publishers
Newbury Park   London   New Delhi

For information address:

SAGE Publications, Inc.
2455 Teller Road
Newbury Park, California 91320

SAGE Publications Ltd.
6 Bonhill Street
London EC2A 4PU
United Kingdom

SAGE Publications India Pvt. Ltd.
M-32 Market
Greater Kailash I
New Delhi 110 048 India

Printed in the United States of America

Library of Congress Cataloging-in-Publication Data

Evans, Christina L. S.
  Imogene King : a conceptual framework for nursing / Christina L. Sieloff Evans.
      p.   cm. — (Notes on nursing theories : vol. 2)
  Includes bibliographical references.
  ISBN 0-8039-4579-5 (cl) ISBN 0-8039-4086-6 (pb)
  1. Nursing — Philosophy. I. Title. II. Series.
  RT84.5.E93 1991
610.73'01—dc20   91-28098
                                                            CIP
92 93 94 15 14 13 12 11 10 9 8 7 6 5 4 3 2

Sage Production Editor: Tara S. Mead

Contents

Foreword

Nursing science has come of age. The multiple publications of conceptual systems and theories in nursing have demonstrated advance in the scientific movement in nursing. This book by Christina Sieloff Evans presents my conceptual system from which a theory of goal attainment was derived. The author is well qualified to do this. She has demonstrated very clearly the difference between a conceptual system and a theory derived from it and has displayed a thorough understanding of theory construction and testing in research. In addition, she has shown an understanding of the theory and the use of my nursing process of interactions that lead to transactions and then to goal attainment.

In the past few years, several nurses have published ways in which they have used knowledge of the concepts of the theory and my nursing process in caring for patients. These publications have shown that the theory is useful in caring for patients in critical care units, in oncology units, in psychiatric units, in community health, and in gerontological nursing situations. One group of nurses in Canada published the way they organized all of the nursing diagnoses under the concepts of this theory. Two nurses in Canada published their ideas about how they planned and implemented change in a hospital and used my conceptual system.

Some of the criteria used by accrediting agencies such as Joint Commission of Accreditation for Healthcare Organizations, indicate an expectation that nurses understand the theoretical basis for their practice. Use of a conceptual system and theory such as mine helps nurses meet this criterion. Several nursing departments in medical centers and community hospitals have used this theory to implement theory-based practice. This monograph increases the focus on nursing science.

IMOGENE M. KING, EDD, RN
Professor Emeritus
University of South Florida
Tampa, Florida

Preface

Nurses routinely set goals for, and frequently with, clients. And yet, how often is that process examined from a nursing theory perspective? Dr. Imogene M. King began writing about nursing theory in 1964 and published her first book in 1971. She developed a conceptual framework for nursing and within this framework developed a theory for nursing that focused on the process of mutual goal setting by nurse and client. By developing a systems approach that focused on a holistic view of human beings, Dr. King:

(1) identified concepts of relevance to nursing,
(2) developed and tested the Theory of Goal Attainment, and
(3) developed the Goal Oriented Nursing Record (1981).

The purpose of this book is to provide a descriptive overview of Dr. King's framework and theory. A brief biography of Dr. King will be presented. The origin of her conceptual framework will be discussed and the framework described. Concepts from the proposed metaparadigm for nursing will then be examined. The Theory of Goal Attainment will be presented and the assumptions and hypotheses discussed. Application of the theory to practice and research will be examined. The bibliography will include publications both by and about Dr. King.

—CHRISTINA L. SIELOFF EVANS

Biographical Sketch of the Nurse Theorist: Imogene M. King, EdD, RN

BSN: St. Louis University, St. Louis, Missouri
MSN: St. Louis University
PhD: Education, Teacher's College, Columbia University,
     New York
Past Professor of Nursing: University of South Florida, Tampa
Professor Emeritus: University of South Florida
Member: American Nurses' Association/Florida Nurses' Association/District IV
Board Member: Operation PAR, Inc.
President: Florida Nurses' Foundation

1

Origin of the Conceptual Framework

Imogene King began developing her conceptual framework in 1961 in order to cultivate a master's program in Nursing at Loyola University in Chicago (Ackermann, Brink, Jones, Moody, Perlich, & Prusinski, 1986). As a beginning step, she examined society and identified several trends in health care, many of which are still applicable today: (a) a knowledge explosion, (b) increasing technological advances, (c) changes in the composition of the population, and (d) mobility of employees. The environment was becoming increasingly complex.

Because nurses were, and are, key persons in health care systems, King developed several questions about nursing:

(1) What is the nursing act?
(2) What is the nursing process?
(3) What is the goal of nursing?
(4) Who are nurses, and how are they educated for practice?
(5) How and where is nursing practiced?
(6) Who needs nursing in this society? (King, 1975a, p. 37)

King reviewed the literature in psychology, sociology, and nursing as she searched for the answers to her questions. She identified words that consistently appeared in the nursing literature. Following an analysis of these words, three initial concepts were identified: inter-personal relations, perception, and organization. In addition, one concept was identified as a major component of the other words—energy.

After reviewing the literature, King discussed her findings at con-ferences and with colleagues. Through this process of critical thinking, using inductive and deductive processes, she began developing her framework (King, 1975a).

Conceptual Framework

King's work resulted in the development of a conceptual framework and the Theory of Goal Attainment. Her conceptual framework will be discussed first, followed by a review of her theory.

A conceptual framework differs from a theory in several ways:

(1) A conceptual framework is usually more abstract than a theory and cannot be directly applied to practice situations. A theory may be used to guide practice.
(2) A conceptual framework presents a broad view of an area of inter-est, for example, human interactions. In contrast, a theory presents a narrower view—for example, the goal attainment aspect of nurse-client interactions.
(3) Although both a conceptual framework and a theory contain con-cepts, the linkages between concepts in a theory are more clearly delineated than in a conceptual framework. (Meleis, 1985)

Systems Framework

King utilized a systems framework as the basis for developing her conceptual framework. General systems theory was developed in the early 1930s by a group of individuals to counteract logical positivism and to offer another approach in the search for scientific knowledge (King, 1990). Logical positivism focused on mechanistic relationships—dividing wholes into parts and determining the re-lationships of these parts. General systems theory is concerned with wholes rather than parts (Bertalanffy, 1968). In examining wholes, one does not examine the total of the parts of a system, for the whole is different from this total—a view consistent with nursing's perspective of an individual.

Elements of any system include structure, function, resources, and goals. In attempting to provide a "structure for nursing as a discipline and as a profession" (King, 1989a, p. 151), King developed a systems framework. According to her theory, the structure of a system may be reflected by a person interacting with an environment. Nursing functions include viewing, recognizing, observing and measuring, synthesizing and interpreting, and analyzing. However, these functions are conducted not in a stepwise manner, but simultaneously within the context of the nursing process. Resources involved are of two types: human and material. The goal of the system is health.

King utilized this systems framework to determine that health concerns related to nursing can be grouped into "three dynamic interacting systems: (a) personal systems, (b) interpersonal systems, and (c) social systems" (King, 1989a, p. 151). Figure 1.1 illustrates this relationship. In addition, following a review of the literature, King identified concepts that are relevant to nursing and nursing practice:

- authority
- body image
- communication
- decision making
- growth and development
- interaction
- organization
- perception
- power
- role
- self
- space
- status
- stress
- time
- transaction

The three "systems, along with identified concepts, provide a way of organizing one's knowledge, skills, and values" (King, 1989a, p. 152).

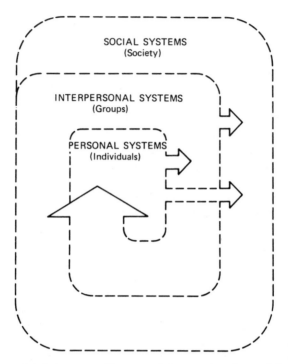

Figure 1.1. A conceptual framework for nursing: dynamic interacting systems. (King 1971, p. 20)

Personal Systems

King conceptualized a personal system as an individual, utilizing information that would assist nurses in understanding individuals. Understanding an individual as a whole is critical before a nurse can understand groups and communities. The concepts of body image, growth and development, perception, self, space, and time are particularly relevant to the personal system.

The personal system focuses on individual human beings. Therefore, it is fitting to discuss King's view of this concept. The concept of a human being is synonymous with that of a personal system within the conceptual framework.

Although King did not define the personal system specifically, she identified several characteristics of a human being. A human being is a complex, open living system that "copes with a wide range of events, persons and things over time" (King, 1975b, p. 6). This human being has the following fundamental health needs: "(a) usable health information at a time when he/she needs it and is able to use it, (b) preventive care, and (c) care when ill" (King, 1971, p. 83).

Human beings are rational and feeling and react to their expectations, other individuals, events, and objects. They react on the basis of their "perceptions, expectations, and needs" (King, 1981, p. 20). They react as a whole, individuals being viewed as an entity, a living system.

Human beings are time-oriented and have an awareness of the past, present, and their future goals. By choosing among alternatives, human beings make decisions. They select goals upon which to focus, and then identify the means to attain them. In addition, a human being, "depending upon habits, abilities, age and situation, has functions to be performed; age, the place in the family, and roles being critical variables" (King, 1975b, p. 6).

Interpersonal Systems

Interpersonal systems focus on groups of individuals, including dyads, triads, or small or large groups. A group's complexity and variability increase concurrent with its size. Concepts more important to interpersonal systems include communication, interaction, roles, stress, and transaction. The interpersonal system is the system in which the nursing process primarily occurs (King, 1981). King (1975a) defined the nursing process as a "series of acts that connote action, reaction, interaction, and transaction between nurse and health client" (p. 37).

Social Systems

A social system is defined by King (1981) as "an organized boundary system of social roles, behaviors and practices developed to maintain values and the mechanisms to regulate the practices and rules" (p. 115). Individuals within a social system share common goals and interests. The social system exists in order to address the specific concerns of these individuals and the subgroups they form within the social system (Gulitz & King, 1988). Families, religions, educational systems, work places, and health care settings are examples of social systems.

All social systems have certain common characteristics. Among these are age gradation, authority, behavior patterns, roles, social interactions, status, structure, and values. However, King (1981) identified the following concepts from the conceptual framework as particularly relevant to a social system: authority, decision making, organization, power, and status.

An individual "functions in social systems through interpersonal relationships in terms of . . . perceptions which influence . . . life and health" (Daubenmire & King, 1973, p. 512). Therefore, it is important for nurses to know about the impact of social systems on individual's and groups' behaviors.

When nursing within a social system, practice focuses on the health needs and wants of a social system. Utilizing the nursing process, a nurse works with individuals and groups within the social system to address the health needs of clients and the wants of the social system. Therefore, "the establishment of mutually set goals, the planning of programs, and the evaluation of outcomes need to focus on the goals of the social system being served" (Gulitz & King, 1988, p. 130).

Assumptions

An assumption is "a statement of principle that is accepted as true on the basis of logic or reason" (Woods & Catanzaro, 1988, p. 552). The following are the original assumptions upon which King's (1971) conceptual framework was based:

(a) Nurses, in the performance of their roles and responsibilities, assist individuals and groups in society to attain, maintain, and restore health.

(b) In the process of functioning in social institutions, nurses assist individuals to meet their basic needs at some point in time in the life cycle when they cannot do this for themselves.

(c) An understanding of basic human needs in the physical, social, emotional, and intellectual realm of the life process from conception to old age, within the context of social systems of the culture in which nurses live and work, is essential and basic content for learning the practice of nursing. (Fawcett, 1984, pp. 88-89)

King states that the 1981 version of her conceptual framework is based on the following assumption: "The focus of nursing is human beings interacting with their environment leading to a state of health for individuals, which is an ability to function in social roles" (Fawcett, 1984, p. 89).

Concepts

Although the concepts of King's (1981) conceptual framework are placed in specific systems, they "are so interrelated in the interactions of human beings with their environment that the placement within each of the three systems is an arbitrary decision" (King, 1989a, p. 151). Thus, each concept is applicable to each of the three dynamic interacting systems (personal, interpersonal, and social) and may be discussed, examined, and utilized within each system. In this section, the concepts have been presented in alphabetical order so that the reader can more easily locate them. These concepts are authority, body image, communication, decision making, growth and development, interaction, organization, perception, power, role, self, space, status, stress, time, and transaction.

The concepts of King's conceptual framework will be presented in a consistent format. This format will include

- title of a concept
- characteristics of, and information regarding, a concept
- an example of the concept

Definitions of the concepts are included in the glossary. Each concept may include one or more of the following types of definitions: (a) conceptual, (b) theoretical from the Theory of Goal Attainment, or (c) operational.

Authority

Authority is the ability "to make decisions that guide the actions of self and others" (King, 1981, p. 122). It may be either formal or functional and is the "legitimate power given to a person by virtue of role and position in a social system" (King, 1981, p. 122). Authority resides in (a) a position that enables an individual to dispense rewards and sanctions, (b) expertise that results from special knowledge and skills, and (c) the leader of a group (King, 1981).

Authority is universal. It is present in every culture and "provides order, guidance, and responsibility for actions" (King, 1981, p. 123). There is a reciprocal relationship between an individual exercising authority and an individual accepting authority. In addition, authority varies with the situation in which it occurs.

In order to function effectively in an organization, nurses need to understand authority. A department of nursing within a health-care organization should have the authority to make nursing-related decisions. To have this authority, nurses within a department need to understand their organizational position and the authority and power related to that position (King, 1981).

Example: A client requested that the bed bath be done later in the morning rather than directly after breakfast. Because the primary nurse was responsible for the completion of the client's care, he had the authority to rearrange the order of that care to meet the client's request.

Body Image

Everyone has a body image, although cultural factors affect the perception of a body image. An individual's body image is personal, subjective, and unique. It cannot be duplicated by another individual. Body image develops over one's life span as input is received regarding the image one, and others, perceive about the body. Thus, body image is dynamic; it changes over time as additional input is received from others and as an individual becomes aware of bodily changes.

Disturbances in one's body image may result from trauma, loss of body parts, or actual or perceived threats to one's person. It is important for a nurse to be aware of a client's perception of body image because the nurse and client work together to develop goals and means to achieve these goals. If a client perceives that a body image may limit the ability to achieve a goal, whether or not this is true, a nurse needs to recognize this perception as real and work with the client in order to provide additional feedback.

An individual's body image is not the only image that affects an individual. The image that family members and friends hold of an individual also influences the individual's perception of body image.

Hence, it is important to include a client's family and friends when addressing goals that involve a client's body image.

Touch contributes to an individual's development of a "healthy body image" (King, 1981, p. 72). Because nurses frequently touch clients while delivering nursing care, it is important that nurses recognize the impact of a client's perception of touch on body image.

Example: A client recently was informed that she has diabetes. Even though there was no overt physical change in her body image, she expressed that she felt ugly and marred. She believed that her body image had been negatively altered.

Communication

Communication occurs through both verbal and nonverbal exchanges. Verbal exchanges can include both spoken and written communications. Nonverbal communication is also extremely important because it provides "accurate information about another person's attitudes and feelings" (King, 1981, p. 71). When the client is unable to verbally communicate, nonverbal communication is a key factor in determining whether or not mutual goal setting occurs. Examples of nonverbal communication include appearance, distance, facial expressions, posture and touch (King, 1981). While communicating, it in important to listen, be silent, and observe how an individual communicates nonverbally.

The interpretation of communication depends upon the situation in which it occurs. Once communication takes place, it cannot be recalled. The impact of communication remains even if subsequent communications attempt to change or eliminate it.

Communication involves the perceptions of both a sender and a receiver. Through communication, transactions may be made between the two individuals (see the discussion on transactions). Each individual's communication is different. No one can say the exact same words in the exact same way with the exact same results.

Communication involves an "interchange of thoughts and opinions among individuals and is a means whereby social interaction and learning take place" (King, 1981, p. 62). Open systems (human beings) continuously communicate through interactions with the environment (King, 1981). This communication may be intrapersonal and primarily nonverbal, or interpersonal (between individuals) and both verbal and nonverbal.

The following factors can influence the "patterns of communication" between individuals: the situation in which the individuals are communicating; the roles, expectations, and goals of each individual, and the barriers to communication (King, 1981).

For communication to be most effective, an environment must exist in which a nurse and a client respect and wish to understand each other. This environment provides motivation for the understanding and utilization of information (King, 1981).

Information "is crucial in the care, cure and recovery" (King, 1981, p. 78) of clients. Thus, communication facilitates the delivery of nursing care because it "establishes a mutuality between care givers and recipients of care" (King, 1981, p. 146). Nurses have the primary responsibility to maintain open communication with the client in order to mutually set goals (King, 1981).

Communication also occurs in nurses' interactions with other nurses, providers, and family members. Hence, it is important that nurses have a knowledge of communication and communication skills (King, 1981).

Example: A nurse observes a comatose client's nonverbal responses to a range of motion exercises. In response to nonverbal communication interpreted negatively by the nurse (e.g. grimaces, frowns), the nurse moves through the exercises more slowly. The nurse and the client have communicated.

Decision Making

Decision making is a personal process that involves subjective behaviors; it is individual. Decision making is also situational because it is affected by the time of the decision, the information available, and the individuals participating (King, 1981). Because each decision results in the need for additional decision-making behaviors, the decision-making process is continuous. Decision making occurs to achieve a goal.

There are three components to every decision: (a) the process, (b) the decision maker, and (c) the resulting decision. Situational variables impact the decision-making process by influencing clients' decisions regarding goal prioritization and the means to achieve these goals (King, 1981). Variables related to a nurse and a client occur as a result of their "knowledge, background of experience, goals, values, and perceptions of the situation" (King, 1981, p. 134).

Participation in decision making leads to decreased resistance to decision implementation, and learning occurs. Decision makers are viewed as having authority and power. Decision making affects the quality of care delivered throughout a health-care setting (King, 1981). Hence, decision making is a key factor in both the delivery of nursing care and in the administrative functions of a department.

Example: After identifying the possible goals available, the nurse and client began to prioritize them. After ranking the goals, they selected one goal. They engaged in decision making.

Growth and Development

Growth and development is a "function of: (a) genetic endowment, (b) meaningful and satisfying experiences, and (c) an environment conducive to helping individuals [and groups] move toward maturity" (King, 1981, p. 31). Growth and development also include behavioral, cellular, and molecular changes.

Age is an important variable in determining an individual's growth and development. The age of a system defines "the stage of each [system's] developmental tasks" (King, 1981, p. 148).

Groups can also experience growth and development, moving from a potential to an actualization of their abilities and goals. Through knowledge of social systems and related concepts, a nurse can assess a group's level of growth and development.

Knowledge of growth and development patterns is useful if nurses are to help clients through stressful periods. Familiarity with the normal patterns of growth and development enables a nurse to identify disruptions in these patterns and to assist clients in establishing goals to alleviate those disruptions.

Example: When completing an admission assessment with a twelve-year-old girl, the nurse assessed the child's developmental and chronological age. The nurse assessed the child's level of growth and development.

Interaction

All human beings and groups interact with values influencing each interaction. When individuals and groups interact, they respond to each other through mutuality—"interdependence in the situation in which both achieve goals" (King, 1981, p. 84). Verbal and nonverbal communication are present in every interaction.

The process of an interaction moves forward; it is unidirectional. Occurring within a time-space context, an interaction is a continuous process. Once an interaction occurs, it cannot be repeated.

Certain factors are to be considered when viewing interactions. These factors include (a) the situation, (b) the context of the interaction, (c) the closeness of the participants, and (d) the interdependency of each person. Inferences are made as a result of an interaction, and their accuracy results from verification with the other person.

> In nursing, the primary purpose of interactions is to assist an individual to cope with a health problem or concern about health. . . . Nurses and [clients] respond through interactions to the humanness of each other, to the presence of each other, and to the reciprocally contingent relationship. Interactions help nurses and [clients] clarify the shared environment. (King, 1981, pp. 85-86)

Purposeful interactions require that nurse and client openly share information and agree on the means to achieve goals. By being open to cues given during an interaction, each participant is more able to process information. Purposeful, goal-oriented interactions in nursing situations also enhance the effectiveness of care and create positive outcomes for those involved (King, 1981).

King (1981) presented the following assumptions about nurse-client interactions:

(1) Perceptions of nurse and of client influence the interaction process.
(2) Goals, needs, and values of nurse and client influence the interaction process.
(3) Individuals have a right to knowledge about themselves.
(4) Individuals have a right to participate in decisions that influence their life, their health, and community services.
(5) Health professionals have a responsibility to share information that helps individuals make informed decisions about their health care.
(6) Individuals have a right to accept or reject health care.
(7) Goals of health professionals and goals of recipients of health care may be incongruent. (King, 1981, pp. 143-144)

Example: A client turned on her call light. The nurse responded by entering the client's room and asking if he could help her. The client responded that she had questions about her discharge plans. The nurse began to answer the client's questions. The nurse and client interacted.

Organization

An organization ensures an arrangement of positions and actions. It has structure. Within this structure, an organization is associated with roles, positions, and actions to be executed; an organization demonstrates function (King, 1981).

All organizations have goals, and resources are utilized for goal achievement. Successful decision making is crucial for an organization to exist and to be productive (King, 1981).

Organizations arrange individuals in a variety of ways that are designed to attain organizational goals (King, 1981). the focus of an organization is to achieve goals. The system view of an organization "emphasizes the design of communication, information flow and decisions" (King, 1981, p. 118). An organization, as a system, connects questions and answers.

Components of an organization include:

(1) human values, behavior patterns, needs, goals and expectations;
(2) a natural environment in which material and human resources are essential for achieving goals;
(3) employers and employees or parents and children, who form groups that collectively interact to achieve goals; and
(4) technology that facilitates goal achievement. (King, 1981, p. 116)

A knowledge of the concept of organization is essential for nurses working within social systems. To function professionally and to achieve quality care standards, nurses must exert influence on an organization (King, 1981).

King (1989b, p. 42) proposed the following criteria for the analysis of an organization:

• the philosophy of the organization
• the goals of the organization
• the structure of the organization

- the functions of the organization
- the resources available to accomplish the goals
- the constraints in the organization
- the clarity of the lines of communication and responsibility
- who makes the decisions

King suggests the following techniques for successful functioning within an organization once the nurse has analyzed the organization, (King, 1981, p. 121):

(1) Assess the organization, using objective criteria, to determine if your professional and personal goals mesh with the organizational goals.
(2) Agree with the written philosophy and its implementation.
(3) Agree with the goals of the organization.
(4) Know who makes decisions that affect care.
(5) Identify the lines of formal and informal communication and the power.
(6) Assess the kind of management that prevails.

Example: A hospital is an organization with a formal structure (organizational plan) and specific functions assigned to designated individuals and groups. Utilizing available resources, individuals and groups focus on achieving goals.

Perception

Every human being perceives, and each person's perceptions are different from those of others. Perception involves the individual taking action at the present time (King, 1981).

Perception is a basic concept (King, 1981). Perception occurs through the use of both "sensory (functioning sense organs) and intellectual (brain processes) tools" (King, 1981, p. 20). Perception is related to an individual's or group's education, experiences, goals, needs, physiology, self concept, socioeconomic status, temporal-spatial relationships, and values (King, 1981).

The perceptual process for open systems (human beings) involves the following elements: "(a) import of energy from the environment organized by information, (b) the transformation of energy, (c) processing of information, (d) storing of information, and (e) export of information in overt behavior" (King, 1981, p. 146).

Perception "gives meaning to one's experience, represents one's image of reality and influences one's behavior, and is the basis for developing a concept of self" (King, 1981, pp. 24-25). Perception enables a human being to know (a) self, (b) others, and (c) "objects in the environment" (King, 1981, p. 19). Reflective of this importance of perception, it is important to note that perception may be distorted by stress and sensory overload or deprivation (King, 1981).

In addition, perceptual congruence is an important element in nurse-client interactions and is the "first step in mutual goal setting" (King, 1981, p. 24). Nurses need to recognize factors that influence perceptions to avoid making inferences on the basis of limited behavioral cues (King, 1981). Hence, by understanding perceptions, nurses can better understand their selves and their clients (King, 1989a).

Example: A client developed an understanding of her upcoming surgery from talking with the physician, the anesthetist and the recovery room nurse. The client's primary nurse identified that this understanding was not accurate because the client believed that she would be able to get out of bed immediately after surgery. The client's perception of what she was told was different from the information that had been provided.

Power

Power is universal and related to a situation, not a person. Because power is situational, and situations change, power also changes. Directed toward the achievement of a goal, the exercise of power within a relationship depends upon the acceptance of power. The existence of power "implies a dependency relationship" (King, 1981, p. 126).

The concepts of authority, influence, and status are related to power. Authority is the "legitimate power given to a person by virtue of role and position in a social system in a formal organization" (King, 1981, p. 123). "Influence is an instance of power in which outcomes are not predetermined" (King, 1981, p. 126). Status can be interpreted as personal power (King, personal communication, 1990).

Power is a characteristic of a social system and is equivalent to energy "in the physical world" (King, 1981, p. 126). Uses of power within a social system include budget control, decision making, information control, and reward/sanction control (King, 1981). Power "protects relationships among people to maintain order and to achieve goals" (King, 1981, p. 128) and is "essential in an organization for the maintenance of balance and harmony" (King, 1981, p. 126). Powe involves a method of obtaining needed resources that facilitate the production of organizational efficiency (King, 1981).

According to King (1981, p. 127), power (a) enhances group cohesive ness, and (b) is a function of human interactions and decision making

"Each person," wrote King "has the potential power . . . which i determined by individual resources and the environmental force encountered" (1981, pp. 127-128). Power results from one's role and position, but it is limited by the amount of resources available and the existence of goals. Without goals, power cannot exist (King, 1981) With power, one can exercise "some control over the process of change in an organization" (King, 1981, p. 127).

Example: A nurse asked a unit clerk to rearrange the multiple test scheduled for a client in order to provide the client with rest periods The nurse utilized his power to rearrange the client's scheduled tests

Roles

Roles are "learned from functioning in a variety of social system within society" (King, 1981, p. 92). Roles are complex and situational Individuals or groups may exchange roles depending on the situation

The concept of roles requires individuals to communicate and t "interact in purposeful ways to achieve goals" (King, 1981, p. 91). The role of a nurse can be defined as an "interaction between one or mor individuals who come to a nursing situation in which nurses perforn functions of professional nursing based on knowledge, skills, and values identified as nursing" (King, 1981, p. 93).

Nurses have both expressive roles, which focus on maintainin balance in a system, and instrumental roles, which focus on action that assist a system in achieving goals. In order for nurses to functio professionally, they must define their role. If employer expectation differ from professional expectations, role conflict will result. Rol conflict may then reduce the effectiveness of nursing care and produc stress. Therefore, a knowledge of the concept of roles is important fo professional nurses (King, 1981).

Example: During the week, a nurse functioned as a primary nurs with a caseload of 5 patients. During weekends, the nurse assume additional managerial responsibilities for the unit. She assumed the role of charge nurse.

Self

The self is an open system. As an individual has new experiences, the self changes to incorporate information from these experiences. An individual or a group "directs activities toward fulfillment of self" (King, 1981, p. 27); the self is goal directed.

"Knowledge of self is a key to understanding human behavior," King wrote (1981, p. 26). Both a nurse and a client have a self. In order for a nurse to assist a client, the nurse must understand the client's self-perception (King, 1981). If a nurse facilitates the ability of an individual or a group to be true to the self, both the nurse and the individual or group "grow in self-awareness and in understanding of human behavior" (King, 1981, p. 28).

Example: A client who was short and underweight acted as if he were tall and muscular. The nurse, recognizing the client's perception of self, responded to the perception, not the physical appearance.

Space

Space is a "function of area, volume, distance and . . . time" (King, 1981, p. 37). Space exists within all cultures but is perceived differently by each individual and depends upon the situation (King, 1981). "Space determines the transactions between human beings and the environment" (King, 1981, p. 37).

Space is an essential component in an open-system framework. Knowledge of space is important for nurses to understand both their own and a client's self in relation to personal space. Because personal space is associated with self identity, it is relevant when considering the distance involved in providing personal care to patients (King, 1981).

Example: When a nurse came too close to the newly admitted client, the client's muscles tensed. By increasing the personal space of the client, the nurse facilitated the client's relaxation.

Status

An individual's or group's status depends upon the situation in which that individual or group exists. Status also depends on the position held within a situation. Because status is related to a position, the level of status can decrease when a position is changed.

Status can be considered as the "prestige attached to a role [and is] associated with individuals [or groups] who have the power and authority to make decisions" (King, 1981, pp. 129-130). Because these decisions often influence the attainment of client care goals, departments of nursing should have equal status with all other departments. Thus, it is important for nurses to recognize the significance of status in the process of goal attainment (King, 1981).

Example: Within the health care setting, a nurse who has conducted research is perceived as more valuable to the Director of Nursing than are other nurses. This nurse has status.

Stress

All human beings experience stress, and the level of stress experienced by an individual or group constantly changes. Stress is experienced by human beings in a personal and subjective manner and "is not limited by time or place" (King, 1981, p. 97).

King views stress as an energy response of an individual to persons, objects, and events called "stressors" (1981, p. 99). The level of stress experienced by an individual is influenced by a variety of factors. Individual or group factors include, but are not limited to:

- age
- cognition
- environmental background
- meaning of the event
- motivation
- personality
- response
- sex/predominant gender (group)
- situation
- stressors
- the time of the event (King, 1981)

An increase in stress lowers one's ability both to perceive events and to make rational decisions (King, 1981). This "may then lead to decreased interactions and goal setting between nurse and [client], and to ineffective nursing care. In addition, subsequent interference in each person's developmental tasks may occur" (King, 1981, p. 148). Nurses can decrease stress through various techniques, which may include:

(1) providing information,
(2) assessing physiological change,
(3) assisting clients (individuals or groups) to articulate concerns,
(4) facilitating goal setting by clients (individuals or groups), and
(5) suggesting alternative means to attain the goals. (King, 1981)

Example: At the change of shift—a busy time for nurses—two clients were admitted. Arriving when they did, these admissions added stress to the nurses involved.

Time

Time is universal and exists in every culture. However, time is based on an individual's perceptions of the movement of life events (King, 1981).

"Time moves from the past to the future" (King, 1981, p. 43) and is measurable. However, time is to be viewed in relation to other concepts such as age, body temperature, order of events, sequence of events, and space.

There are several time perspectives: (a) biological, (b) psychological, which is perceived subjectively, (c) physical, as measured by clocks, and (d) relational, which connects the past with the present and the future. However, time is defined by each individual (King, 1981).

Example: Within 5 minutes, the nurse returned to the client with a pain medication. To the client, it seemed as though half an hour had passed. Each had a different perception of time.

Transaction

The concept of transaction was developed from a review of research literature that identified its characteristics. From these characteristics, a definition was formulated. A transaction involves the perceptions of individuals and is therefore unique. It concerns both verbal and non-verbal communication. Each transaction is a "series of events in time" used to achieve a goal (King, 1981, pp. 80-81).

Whereas communication is the informational component of inter-actions, transaction is the "valuational component" (King, 1981, p. 62). Transaction "involves bargaining, negotiating, and social exchange, and is influenced by role expectations and role performance" (King, 1981, p. 147).

A transaction "represents a life situation in which . . . each person enters the situation as an active participant, and each is changed in the process of these experiences"(King, 1981, p. 142). A transaction is affected by the actions, judgments, perceptions, and reactions of human beings (King, 1981). The "unit of analysis is the dyadic inter-actions of nurse and [client] who come together in a specific place called a nursing situation that is within a larger system called a health care system" (King, 1981, p. 83).

Goal attainment occurs as a result of a transaction between a nurse and a client (King, 1981). Transaction involves the process of mutual goal setting and the joint establishment of the means to achieve the goal.

Example: A nurse and a client discussed how they could work together to decrease the client's use of pain medications. They decide that the goal would be 2 pain pills per 24-hour period. They identified relaxation techniques that could be utilized to increase the length of time between pain pills and determined that they would increase the length of time between pain pills by half an hour each time. Together, they implemented this plan until, on the third day, the client was comfortable with only two pain pills in 24 hours.

Metaparadigm Concepts

Metaparadigm concepts identified in the nursing literature are: (a) environment, (b) health, (c) nursing, and (d) person. Although there is controversy as to whether nursing should be included as a metaparadigm concept, the following section reviews King's writings about 3 of these 4 concepts. (Person was discussed in relation to personal systems.)

Health

Each culture defines health differently. King's definition of health is "a dynamic state of an individual in which change is [a] constant and an ongoing process" (1989a, p. 152); it is a "functional state in the life cycle" (King, 1981, p. 5).

According to King (1981, p. 4), health is a "process of human growth and development [and] relates to the way individuals deal with the stress of growth and development while functioning within the cultural pattern in which they were born and to which they attempt to conform." Health is needed in order to lead a "useful, satisfying, productive and happy life. The level of health depends on harmony and balance in each person's environment" (King, 1981, p. 4).

Health and illness are not part of a linear continuum. King has chosen not to address wellness because it is too abstract and would lend support to the continuum perspective (King, 1990). Whereas health is a "functional state in the life cycle, [illness is] some interference in the cycle" (King, 1981, p. 5). King defines illness as a "deviation from normal, that is, an imbalance in a person's biological structure or . . . psychological make-up, or a conflict in a person's social relationship" (1981, p. 5).

Preventing illness is not the same as promoting health. Health of individuals and groups is "the goal for nursing" (King, 1975b, p. 37).

Environment

King does not discuss environment directly in her 1981 book. However, she does define the environment as the social system surrounding the concept in question (1990). Hence, the environment of a child could include family, school, peer, religious, and neighborhood social systems.

In addition, King determined that an environment can be both external and internal. In this holistic view of the environment, external and internal aspects are interrelated. For example, the "internal environment of human beings transforms energy to enable them to adjust to continuous external environmental changes" (King, 1981, p. 5).

Nursing

Nursing involves (a) "recognition of presenting conditions, (b) operations or activities related to the situation or conditions, and (c) motivation to exert some control over the events in the situation to achieve goals" (King, 1981, p. 144). Goal setting occurs in every nursing situation (King, 1981). Other important aspects of nursing are (a) listening, (b) communicating, (c) special knowledge, (d) professional skills and values, and (e) goal setting (King, 1981).

King (1989a, p. 150) wrote that the focus of nursing is the interaction of human beings with their environment "in ways that lead to self fulfillment and to maintenance of health" (1981, p. 3)—the "care of human beings" (1981, p. 10). What makes nursing unique, according to King (1981), is the way nurses use knowledge to perform their functions. Nursing goals are separate from the activities undertaken to attain them, and they are "distinct from the goals of other professions" (King, 1981, p. 97).

King defines the domain of nursing as promotion, maintenance, and restoration of health, and care of the sick, injured, and dying (1981). The goal of nursing is to "help individuals maintain their health so they can function in their roles" (King, 1981, pp. 3-4).

The function of nursing is, in King's view, to "teach, guide and counsel individuals and groups to help them maintain health" (1981, p. 8). This function includes the "interpretation of specific information to plan, implement and evaluate nursing care. Knowledge from natural and behavioral sciences and the humanities is integrated and applied in concrete situations" (King, 1981, p. 8). This knowledge is applied in relation to human behavior under normal and stressful conditions. Techniques used by nurses include (a) assessment, (b) communication, (c) systematic gathering of information, (d) interviews, (e) measurement, and (f) observation.

The basic unit of nursing behavior is a nursing act; an interaction between a nurse and client (King, 1989a). These interactions focus on the concerns of the client (King, 1981). It is "important to move toward reciprocally contingent interactions where the behavior of one person influences the behavior of the other, . . . which requires participation by both individuals" (King, 1981, p. 85). A nurse is responsible for initiating a relationship with a client. While attempting to understand a client's behavior, a nurse involves the client in decision making and provides information for determining means to achieve goals. Nurses must be aware of a client's right to make decisions, and must provide information in order for clients to make informed choices (King, 1981). While a nurse assists a client in better understanding the perception of self and "what is happening to interfere with life events, both {the nurse and the client} help each other increase their coping behavior, and they grow in the process" (King, 1981, p. 87).

There are essential variables in nursing situations. These include communication, expectations, interdependent roles of a nurse and client, location, mutual goals, and perceptions (King, 1981).

Propositions

A proposition is a statement that "identifies a relationship between concepts" (Catanzaro & Woods, 1988, p. 20). Although distinct relationships between concepts are not always distinguished within a conceptual framework, the following propositions were initially identified by King (1964). To assist the reader, concepts from the conceptual framework and metaparadigm have been italicized.

- The *nursing* process is conducted within a *social system*. The dimensions include: 1) *nursing* process, 2) the *individuals* involved in the *nursing* process, 3) the *individuals* involved in the *environment* within which the *nursing* process is activated, 4) the social organization within which the *nursing* process is activated, [and] 5) the community within which the social organization functions.
- The *nursing* process will differ, dependent upon the individual nurse and each recipient of *nursing* service.
- The *nursing* process will differ relative to all *individuals* in the *environment*.
- The *nursing* process will differ relative to the social organization in which the *nursing* process takes place.
- The relationships among the dimensions have an effect upon the *nursing* process.
- *Nursing* includes specific components: 1) *nursing* judgment, 2) nurse action, 3) *communication*, 4) evaluation, [and] 5) coordination.
- The *nursing* judgment will vary relative to each *nursing* action.
- The effectiveness of *nursing* action will vary with the extent to which it is *communicated* to those responsible for its implementation.

- *Nursing* action is more effectively assured if the goals are *communicated* and standards of *nursing* performance have been established.
- *Nursing* action is based on facts, which may change; thus, *nursing* judgments and action are evaluated and revised as the situation changes.
- *Nursing* is a component of *health* care; thus, *health* care is effected by the coordination of *nursing* with *health* services. (pp. 401-402)

2

Theory of Goal Attainment

King has derived one theory from her conceptual framework—the Theory of Goal Attainment. The focus of this theory is the interpersonal system because what nurses do with, and for, individuals is what "makes the difference between nursing and any other health profession. [The focus of the theory is on] holism—that is, the total human being interacting with another total human being in a specific situation" (King, 1989a, pp. 154-155).

The Theory of Goal Attainment is a "theory of nursing [that] deals with phenomena called process and outcome" (Smith, 1988, p. 82). The process that is the critical, independent variable is mutual goal setting. The theory "defines outcomes in the form of the goals to be attained" (King, 1989a, p. 156). If the goals are identified as client behaviors, then they become criteria by which the effectiveness of nursing care can be measured (King, 1989a).

Context

King characterized the context within which the Theory of Goal Attainment occurs as:

(a) Nurse and client do not know each other.
(b) Nurse is licensed to practice professional nursing.

(c)   Client is in need of the services provided by the nurse.

(d)   Nurse and client are in a reciprocal relationship in that the nurse has special knowledge and skills to communicate appropriate information to help client set goals. Client has information about self and perceptions of problems or concerns that, when communicated to nurse, will help in mutual goal setting.

(e)   Nurse and client are in mutual presence, purposefully interacting to achieve goals.

(f)   Interactions are in a two-person group.

(g)   Interactions are limited to licensed professional nurse and to a client in need of nursing care.

(h)   Interactions are taking place in natural environments. (King, 1981, p. 150)

Assumptions

The following are the assumptions on which the Theory of Goal Attainment is based:

(a)   Individuals are social beings.

(b)   Individuals are sentient beings.

(c)   Individuals are rational beings.

(d)   Individuals are reacting beings.

(e)   Individuals are perceiving beings.

(f)   Individuals are controlling beings.

(g)   Individuals are purposeful beings.

(h)   Individuals are action-oriented beings.

(i)   Individuals are time-oriented beings.

(j)   Perceptions of nurse and of client influence the interaction process.

(k)   Goals, needs and values of nurse and client influence the interaction process.

(l)   Individuals have a right to knowledge about themselves.

(m)   Individuals have a right to participate in decisions that influence their life, their health, and community services.

(n)   Health professionals have a responsibility to share information that helps individuals make informed decisions about their health care.

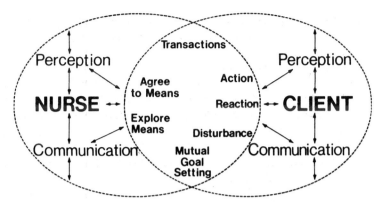

Figure 2.1. Schematic diagram of a theory of goal attainment.
SOURCE: King, 1981, p. 157. Copyright 1981 by Delmar Publishers, Inc. Reprinted by permission.

(o) Individuals have a right to accept or reject health care.
(p) Goals of health professionals and goals of recipients of health care may be incongruent. (King, 1981, pp. 143-144)

Concepts

Major elements in the theory lie within the interpersonal system "in which two people . . . come together . . . to help and be helped to maintain a state of health that permits functioning in roles" (King, 1981, p. 142). The theory uses the concepts of communication, growth and development, interaction, perception, role, self, space, stress, time, and transaction.

The theory also identifies that "decision making is a shared collaborative process in which client and nurse give information to each other, identify goals, and explore means to attain goals; each moves forward to attain goals" (King, 1989a, p. 155). Figure 2.1 illustrates how goals are attained according to this theory.

The theory cannot be directly applied to practice because of its abstract nature. However, one can apply knowledge of the concepts in practice. If relationships among concepts within practice are identified and tested in research, the resulting knowledge can also then be applied (King, 1989a).

Propositions

The following are the propositions of the Theory of Goal Attainment. To assist the reader, the theory's concepts have been italicized.

(a) If *perceptual* accuracy is present in nurse-client *interactions, trans–actions* will occur.

(b) If nurse and client make *transactions,* goals will be attained.

(c) If goals are attained, satisfactions will occur.

(d) If goals are attained, effective nursing care will occur.

(e) If *transactions* are made in nurse-client *interactions, growth and development* will be enhanced.

(f) If *role* expectations and *role* performance as *perceived* by nurse and client are congruent, *transactions* will occur.

(g) If *role* conflict is experienced by nurse or client or both, *stress* in nurse-client *interactions* will occur.

(h) If nurses with special knowledge and skills *communicate* appropriate information to clients, mutual goal setting and goal attainment will occur. (King, 1981, p. 149)

Testing of the Theory of Goal Attainment

King states that "the first phase of testing the theory was to describe nurse-[client] interactions that lead to transactions in concrete nursing situations" (1981, p. 151). A study was designed to answer 3 questions.

First, "What elements in nurse-[client] interactions lead to transactions?" (King, 1981, p. 151). King's research resulted in the following elements of interactions that may lead to transactions: (a) the client identifies a health concern; (b) the "nurse and [client] explore the situation, share information and mutually set goals" (King, 1981, p. 154); (c) the nurse and client explore means by which the concern can be addressed, the goal attained, thus implementing the plan and achieving the goal.

Question 2 asked, "What are the relationships between the elements in the interactions that lead to transactions?" (King, 1981, p. 151). King defined 6 relationships that were identified as predictors or independent variables (King, 1981). These relationships, or behaviors, are:

(a) one member of the nurse-client dyad initiates behavior;

(b) opposite member of the nurse-client dyad responds with behavior;

(c) disturbance (or problem) is noted in the dyadic situation if a state or condition is identified;

(d) some goal is mutually agreed upon by members of the dyad;

(e) exploration of means to achieve goals is initiated by one member of dyad, or behavior is exhibited by member of dyad that moves toward goals; [and]

(f) other member agrees with means to achieve goal. (King, 1981, pp. 150-151)

The presence of these behaviors could predict the possibility of transactions. The seventh behavior was labeled as the dependent variable.

The third question asked was, "What are the essential variables in nurse-[client] interactions that result in transactions?" (King, 1981, p. 151). As a result of the research, the following variables are proposed as essential in nurse-[client] interactions. The first variable is that the perceptions regarding the situation of both a nurse and a client need to be congruent. The perceptions could relate to expectations, goals, health concerns, means to achieve goals, and roles. Relevant communication also must be present. Finally, if a transaction is to occur, mutual goal setting must be present. Together, a nurse and client collaborate in identifying goals to be achieved. For additional details about the method, procedure, sample, and outcome of the study, see King, 1981, pages 153-156.

Hypotheses

The hypotheses of a theory are "tentative statements that can be tested empirically" (Woods & Catanzaro, 1988, p. 558). Dr. King derived the following hypotheses from the Theory of Goal Attainment:

(a) Perceptual accuracy in nurse-[client] interactions increases mutual goal setting.

(b) Communication increases mutual goal setting between nurses and [clients] and leads to satisfactions.

(c) Satisfactions in nurses and [clients] increase goal attainment.

(d) Goal attainment decreases stress and anxiety in nursing situations.

(e) Goal attainment increases [client] learning and coping ability in nursing situations.

(f) Role conflict experienced by [clients], nurses, or both decreases transactions in nurse-[client] interactions.

(g) Congruence in role expectations and role performance increases transactions in nurse-[client] interactions. (1981, p. 156)

The following additional hypotheses have been developed and tested by other researchers:

(1) Functional abilities will be greater in clients who participate in mutual goal setting than in clients who do not.

(2) Goal attainment will be greater with clients who participate in mutual goal setting than with clients who do not.

(3) There will be a positive relationship between a client's functional abilities and goal attainment.

(4) Mutual goal setting will increase a client's functional abilities in activities of daily living.

(5) Mutual goal setting will increase elderly clients' morale.

(6) Mutual goal setting by client and nurse leads to goal attainment.

(7) Mutual goal setting by client and nurse leads to increased satisfaction for both.

(8) Mutual goal setting increases self esteem of the client. (King, 1990)

3

Utilization of the Conceptual Framework and the Theory of Goal Attainment

Whereas the conceptual framework provides nurses with a perspective from which to practice, the "Theory of Goal Attainment provides a theoretical base for nursing process as it demonstrates a way for nurses to interact purposefully with clients" (King, 1981, p. 176). Both the conceptual framework and the theory can be applied to various nursing contexts. These applications include

- assisting nurses to arrange facts into meaningful wholes
- developing research hypotheses
- providing a foundation for nursing care administration
- developing curriculum
- practice applications (King, 1989a)
- delineating the Goal Oriented Nursing Record
- measuring the effectiveness of nursing care through quality assurance activities (King, 1981)

The following uses of the conceptual framework and the Theory of Goal Attainment in nursing practice will be discussed:

(1) use of the conceptual framework to guide the nursing process,

(2) use of the theory related to the Goal Oriented Nursing Record (GONR), and

(3) the Criterion-Referenced Measure of Goal Attainment.

Nursing Process

The following discussion describes the nursing process as it could be conducted according to King's (1981) conceptual framework. In the assessment phase of the nursing process, nurses gather information about a nurse, a client, and a situation. To do this, nurses employ observation and measurement skills (King, 1989a). An assessment could include the following information that has been arranged based on King's (1981) framework:

(1) body image

(2) growth and development
  (a) chronological age
  (b) developmental age
  (c) diet history
  (d) education
  (e) medication history
  (f) initial assessment of a client's intact sensory system
  (g) interference in any of the senses
  (h) sex
  (i) substance abuse history

(3) perceptions
  (a) anxiety level
  (b) current health status
  (c) reason for seeking health care
  (d) stress level

(4) self
  (a) communication style between client and family, and client and health care providers
  (b) culture
  (c) learning needs

     (d) motivation for learning

     (e) space

     (f) personal space definition

  (5) time

     (a) time orientation

     (b) time estimation (King, 1981)

In the planning phase of nursing, a nurse determines client needs by communicating (verbally and nonverbally), observing, and interpreting information (King, 1981). A nurse and a client engage in mutual goal setting and identification of the means to achieve them.

Implementation occurs when a nurse and client work together in a unique relationship in a health care setting. In this relationship, a client has an active role in making decisions about the present and future and gains control and independence through this participation (King, 1981). Together, a nurse and client begin to implement mechanisms by which the mutually agreed upon goals can be attained, and the needs of a client can be met. For example, a client's need for personal space could be met by a nurse (a) controlling the client care environment, (b) explaining to a client why a nurse was in that client's room, (c) explaining procedures prior to their implementation, and (d) orienting a client to the health care setting (King, 1981).

Evaluation occurs when a nurse and client determine whether or not the mutually set goals were attained. Goals may then be revised, or new goals mutually established, to continue the process.

Goal Oriented Nursing Record (GONR)

The GONR records both the process (means utilized to achieve goals) and the outcomes (attainment of goals) (King, 1981). This documentation system demonstrates that quality assurance in nursing includes process and outcomes based on the Theory of Goal Attainment. The GONR has five major elements: data base, nursing diagnoses, goal lists, nursing orders that accompany the goals, plans, and progress notes.

The data base contains all assessment information regarding an individual client. Based on the information in the data base, a nurse develops nursing diagnoses. These diagnoses are revised as they are resolved and as new information is obtained. The diagnoses serve as a guide for "continual assessment of subjective and objective signs and symptoms of a disturbance or interference in clients' ability to perform in usual roles, . . . [and] planning the immediate nursing care" (King, 1981, p. 170).

The goal list results from nurse-client interactions that focus on plans for the resolution of previously identified concerns. In addition, the goal list can serve several purposes:

(1) Assist a nurse in monitoring the health concerns of a client.
(2) Serve as a mechanism for a nurse and client to transact.
(3) Foster the provision of continuity of care.
(4) Emphasize a client's involvement in health care decisions.
(5) "Provide a consistent and systematic approach to help individuals move toward a healthy state.
(6) Facilitate nursing audits" (King, 1981, p. 171).

The plan is founded on the data base. It includes the nursing diagnoses, goals, and actions utilized by the nurse and client to achieve those goals (King, 1981).

Progress notes provide the documentation of the nursing care and client involvement. Progress notes can be one of the following 3 types: (a) narrative, (b) flow sheet (could be designed like a table for the presentation of data) (King, 1990), and (c) final summary or discharge note that describes the status of the goals.

Criterion-Referenced Measure of Goal Attainment (CRMGA)

Another application of the Theory of Goal Attainment to nursing practice is the Criterion-Referenced Measure of Goal Attainment (CRMGA). This measure estimates a client's "functional ability and goal attainment, [developed] to measure goal attainment . . . in nursing situations" (King, 1988, p. 198).

Nurses generally establish goals. However, they "have not always stated them in terms of expected client performance behavior that is observable and/or measureable" (King, 1988, p. 110). There are 3 objectives for the instrument related to a client's performance of daily living activities: a) "assess physical ability of individuals . . . , b) assess the behavioral response of individuals . . . , and c) select a goal and measure goal attainment" (King, 1988, p. 111).

There are 3 scales in the instrument: physical abilities, behavioral responses, and goals. Each scale has 3 subscales: personal hygiene, movement, and human interactions.

Some initial reliability and validity estimates of the instrument have been obtained. Interrater reliability was established at 85% within a nursing home setting and 99% in a critical care setting (King, 1988). (For additional data regarding the reliability and validity estimates, refer to King, 1988.)

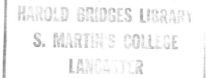

4

Future Directions for Research

As evidenced by the hypotheses previously detailed, research about King's conceptual framework and Theory of Goal Attainment is ongoing. However, much work remains to be done. King has indicated (1990) that additional research should focus on the application of her theory to school, home health practice, occupational health, and transcultural settings. Additional research that uses the conceptual framework to develop theories within the three systems (personal, interpersonal, and social) would also aid in extending the application of King's work.

5

Summary

King's conceptual framework and theory focus on the mutual presence of a nurse and a client as they work together regarding the client's health concerns. By viewing both the nurse and client holistically, an emphasis is placed on verbal and nonverbal communication. As a nurse and client mutually set client goals and the means to achieve these goals, the focus remains on a client's active involvement in health care.

King's conceptual framework and theory can be used to develop: (1) theory-based clinical nursing practice, (2) nursing administration within a social systems context, (3) nursing curriculums, (4) nursing knowledge, and (5) nursing theories. "The value of viewing nursing within this general system framework is a special way of looking at phenomena—holistically," wrote King, "yet within a specific focus based on the situation" (1989a, p. 154).

Glossary

Authority
Conceptual Framework: "transactional process characterized by active reciprocal relations in which members' values, backgrounds, and perceptions play a role in defining, validating, and accepting the [directions] of individuals within an organization" (King, 1981, p. 124)

Body Image
Conceptual Framework: "an individual's perceptions of his/her own body, others' reactions to his/her appearance which results from others' reactions to self" (King, 1981, p. 33).

Communication
Conceptual Framework: "information processing, a change of information from one state to another" (King, 1981, p. 69).

Theoretical: "process whereby information is given from one person to another either directly in face-to-face meetings or indirectly through telephone, television, or the written word" (King, 1981, p. 146).

Decision Making
Conceptual Framework: "dynamic and systematic process by which a goal-directed choice of perceived alternatives is made, and acted upon by individuals or groups to answer a question and attain a goal" (King, 1981, p. 132).

Growth and Development
Conceptual Framework: "the processes that take place in an individual's life that help the individual move from potential capacity for achievement to self actualization" (King, 1981, p. 31).

Theoretical: "continuous changes in individuals at the cellular, molecular, and behavioral levels of activities" (King, 1981, p. 148).

Health
Conceptual Framework: "dynamic life experiences of a human being which implies continued adjustment to stressors in the internal and external environment through optimum use of one's resources to achieve maximum potential for daily living" (King, 1981, p. 5).

Interaction
Conceptual Framework: "acts of two or more persons in mutual presence" (King, 1981, p. 85).

Theoretical: "process of perception and communication between person and environment and between person and person, represented by verbal and nonverbal behaviors that are goal-directed" (King, 1981, p. 145).

Nursing
Conceptual Framework: "process of action, reaction, and interaction whereby nurse and client share information about their perceptions in the nursing situation. A nursing situation is the immediate environment, spatial and temporal reality, in which nurse and client establish a relationship to cope with health states and adjust to changes in activities of daily living if the situation demands adjustment" (King, 1981, p. 2).

Theoretical: "process of human interactions between nurse and client whereby each perceives the other and the situation; and through communication, they set goals, explore means, and agree on means to achieve goals" (King, 1981, p. 144).

Organization
Conceptual Framework: "a system whose continuous activities are conducted to achieve goals" (King, 1981, p. 119).

Operational: "composed of human beings with prescribed roles and positions who use resources to accomplish personal and organizational goals" (King, 1981, p. 119).

Perception
Conceptual Framework: "process of organizing, interpreting, and trans forming information from sense data and memory" (King, 1981, p. 24

Theoretical: "each person's representation of reality; awareness of per sons, objects, and events" (King, 1981, p. 146).

Power
Conceptual Framework: "capacity to use resources in organizations t achieve goals"; "process whereby one or more persons influence othe persons in a situation"; "capacity or ability of a group to achieve goals (King, 1981, p. 124).

Role
Conceptual Framework/Theoretical: "set of behaviors expected whe occupying a position in a social system" (King, 1981, p. 93).

Self
Conceptual Framework: "the self is a composite of thoughts and feeling which constitute a person's awareness of his/her individual existenc his/her conception of who and what he/she is. A person's self is th sum total of all he/she can call his/hers. The self includes, among othe things, a system of ideas, attitudes, values and commitments. The se is a person's total subjective environment. It is a distinctive center experience and significance. The self constitutes a person's inner worl as distinguished from the outer world consisting of all other peopl and things. The self is the individual as known to the individual. It that to which we refer when we say 'I' " (Jersild, 1952, pp. 9-10).

Space
Conceptual Framework: "existing in all directions and is the same e erywhere" (King, 1981, p. 37).

Theoretical: "the immediate environment in which nurse and clier interact and move to goal attainment" (King, 1981, p. 149).

Status
Conceptual Framework: "the position of an individual in a group or group in relation to other groups in an organization" (King, 198 p. 129).

Stress
Conceptual Framework/Theoretical: "dynamic state whereby a huma being interacts with the environment to maintain balance for growt

development, and performance which involves an exchange of energy and information between the person and the environment for regulation and control of stressors" (King, 1981, p. 98).

Time
Conceptual Framework: "duration between the occurrence of one event and the occurrence of another event" (King, 1981, p. 44).

Theoretical: "sequence of events moving onward to the future" (King, 1981, p. 148).

Transaction
Conceptual Framework: "process of interaction in which human beings communicate with the environment to achieve goals that are values" (King, 1981, p. 82).

Theoretical: "observable behaviors of human beings interacting with their environment" (King, 1981, p. 147).

Operational: "one member of the nurse-patient dyad initiates behavior. Opposite member of the nurse-patient dyad responds with behavior. Disturbance (or problem) is noted in the dyadic situation if a state or condition is identified. Some goal is mutually agreed upon by members of the dyad. Exploration of means to achieve goals is initiated by one member of dyad, or behavior is exhibited by member of dyad that moves toward goals. Other member agrees with means to achieve goal. Both move toward goal" (King, 1981, pp. 150-151).

References

Ackermann, M. L., Brink, S. A., Jones, C. G., Moody, S. L., Perlich, G. L., & Prusinski, B. B. (1986). Imogene King: Theory of goal attainment. In A. Marriner (Ed.), *Nursing theorists and their work* (pp. 231-245). St. Louis: C. V. Mosby.

Bertalanffy, L. von (1968). *General system theory: Foundations, development, applications.* New York: George Braziller.

Catanzaro, M., & Woods, N. F. (1988). Developing nursing theory. In N. F. Woods & M. Catanzaro (Eds.), *Nursing research: Theory and practice* (pp. 18-34). St. Louis: C. V. Mosby.

Daubenmire, M. J., & King, I. M. (1973). Nursing process models: A systems approach. *Nursing Outlook, 21*(8), 512-517.

Fawcett, J. (1984). *Analysis and evaluation of conceptual models of nursing.* Philadelphia: F. A. Davis.

Gulitz, E. A., & King, I. M. (1988). King's general systems model: Application to curriculum development. *Nursing Science Quarterly, 1*(3), 128-132.

Jersild, A. T. (1952). *In search of self.* New York: Teachers College Press.

King, I. M. (1964, October). Nursing theory: Problems and prospects. *Nursing Science,* 394-403.

King, I. M. (1971). *Toward a theory for nursing: General concepts of human behavior.* New York: John Wiley.

King, I. M. (1975a). A process for developing concepts for nursing through research. In P. J. Verhovick (Ed.), *Nursing research I* (pp. 25-43). Boston: Little, Brown.

King, I. M. (1975b). Patient aspects. In L. J. Shuman, R. D. Speas, Jr., & J. P. Young (Eds.), *Operations research in health care: A critical analysis* (pp. 3-20). Baltimore: The Johns Hopkins University Press.

King, I. M. (1981). *A theory for nursing: Systems, concepts, process.* New York: John Wiley.

King, I. M. (1988). Measuring health goal attainment in patients. In C. F. Waltz & O. L. Strickland (Eds.), *Measurement of nursing outcomes: Measuring client outcomes* (Vol. 1, pp. 108-127). New York: Springer.

King, I. M. (1989a). King's general systems framework and theory. In J. P. Riehl-Sisca (Ed.), *Conceptual models for nursing practice* (3rd ed., pp. 149-158). Norwalk, CT: Appleton & Lange.

King, I. M. (1989b). King's systems framework for nursing administration. In B. Henry, C. Arndt, M. Di Vincenti, & A. Marriner-Tomey (Eds.), *Dimensions of nursing administration: Theory, research, education, practice* (pp. 35-45). Cambridge: Blackwell Scientific Publications.

King, I. M. (1990, July). Speech presented at the Wayne State University College of Nursing Summer Research Conference, Detroit, MI.

Meleis, A. I. (1985). *Theoretical nursing: Development and progress.* Philadelphia: J. B. Lippincott.

Smith, M. J. (1988). Perspectives on nursing science. *Nursing Science Quarterly, 1*(2), 80-85.

Woods, N. F., & Catanzaro, M. (1988). *Nursing research: Theory and practice.* St. Louis: C. V. Mosby.

Bibliography

Other Publications by Imogene King

1964, October. Nursing theory: Problems and prospects. *Nursing Science*, 394-403.
1968. A conceptual frame of reference for nursing. *Nursing Research, 17*(1), 27-31.
1971. *Toward a theory for nursing: General concepts of human behavior.* New York: John Wiley.
1976. The health care systems: Nursing intervention subsystem. In H. H. Werley, A. Zuzich, M. Zajkowski, & A. D. Zagornik (Eds.), *Health research: The systems approach* (pp. 50-51). New York: Springer.
1978. The "why" of theory development. In *Theory development: What, why, how?* (pp. 11-16). New York: National League for Nursing.
1982. The effect of structured and unstructured pre-operative teaching: A replication. *Nursing Research, 31*(6), 324-329.
1984. Effectiveness of nursing care: Use of a goal oriented nursing record in end stage renal disease. *American Association of Nephrology Nurses and Technicians Journal, 11*(2), 11-17, 60.
1987. King's theory of goal attainment. In R. R. Parse (Ed.), *Nursing science: Major paradigms, theories, and critiques* (pp. 107-113). Philadelphia: W. B. Saunders.
1988. Concepts: Essential elements of theories. *Nursing Science Quarterly, 1*(1), 22-25.
1990. Health: The goal for nursing. *Nursing Science Quarterly, 3*(3), 123-128.

Publications About Imogene King

Austin, J. K., & Champion, V. L. (1983). King's theory for nursing: Explication and evaluation. In P. L. Chinn (Ed.), *Advances in nursing theory development* (pp. 49-61). Rockville, MD: Aspen Systems Corporation.

Brown, S. T., & Lee, B. T. (1980). Imogene King's conceptual framework: A proposed model for continuing nursing education. *Journal of Advanced Nursing, 5*(5), 467-473.

Elberson, K. (1989). Applying King's model to nursing administration. In B. Henry, C. Arndt, M. Di Vincenti, & A. Marriner-Tomey (Eds.), *Dimensions of nursing administration: Theory, research, education, practice* (pp. 47-53). Cambridge: Blackwell Scientific Publications.

Fawcett, J. (1984). *Analysis and evaluation of conceptual models of nursing.* Philadelphia: F. A. Davis.

George, J. B. (1985). Imogene M. King. In J. B. George (Ed.), *Nursing theories: The base for professional nursing practice* (pp. 235-256). Englewood Cliffs, NJ: Prentice-Hall.

Gonot, R. J. (1983). Imogene M. King: A theory for nursing. In J. Fitzpatrick & A. Whall (Eds.), *Conceptual models of nursing: Analysis and application.* Bowie, MD: Robert J. Brady.

Hanchett, E. S. (1988). *Nursing frameworks and community as client: Bridging the gap.* Norwalk, CT: Appleton & Lange.

Hanucharurnkul, S. (1989). Comparative analysis of Orem's and King's theories. *Journal of Advanced Nursing, 14*(5), 365-372.

Meleis, A. I. (1985). *Theoretical nursing: Development and progress.* Philadelphia: J. B. Lippincott.

Pearson, A., & Vaughan, B. (1986). *Nursing models for practice.* London: Heinemann Nursing.

Torres, G. (1986). *Theoretical foundations of nursing.* Norwalk, CT: Appleton-Century-Crofts.

About the Author

Christina L. Sieloff Evans, RN, MSN, CNA, received her BSN in 1970 from Wayne State University's College of Nursing, Detroit, Michigan. In 1977, she returned to Wayne State for her MSN (major: Nursing Administration; minor: Psychiatric/Mental Health Nursing with Children and Adolescents). At the time of publication, she is a doctoral student in nursing at the same university. The focus of her dissertation will be the development of an instrument to estimate a nursing department: power. This instrument will be developed to test her theory of departmental system power that was conceptualized following Dr. King's framework.

Certified by ANA as a Nurse Administrator, Ms. Sieloff is the Clinical Director of an in-patient adult psychiatric unit at Oakland General Hospital, Madison Heights, Michigan. A member of the Detroit District of the Michigan Nurses' Association, American Nurses' Association, she is active at the district, state, and national levels. She is also a member of Sigma Theta Tau and the Wayne State University Alumni Association and has written several publications that focus on psychiatric nursing and nursing administration.